The Ayurveda Hair Loss Cure

Preventing Hair Loss and Reversing Healthy Hair Growth For Life Through Proven Ayurvedic Remedies

I0428348

Table of Content

Introduction

My journey with Ayurveda and Anjali began in July 2013. I had been suffering from severe hair loss and very unhealthy hair for the past year. I was already taking some supplements and applying different modern hair loss products but still the hair fall did not abate and seemed to be getting worse. I mentioned this to my friend Anjali and this was the beginning of my voyage to a healthy scalp with beautiful luscious hair.

Anjali Kumar of Bavdhan is an Ayurveda practitioner with a bachelor of Ayurvedic Medicine degree and Surgery in India.

"Ayurveda" is a classical system of medicine founded 5,000 years ago. The word is derived from Sanskrit, the ancient Indian language, and translates into "knowledge of life,"

Ayurveda provides recommendations regarding food, lifestyle and traditional remedies so that healthy people will remain strong and healthy and sick people will improve their symptoms and wellbeing. Ayurveda achieves such great success in healing by harmonizing mind, body and spirit.

I am 39 years old. My hair had constantly been falling over the past year and appeared to accelerated at a shockingly rate. I started coloring my gray hair with store bought expensive permanent color when I was only in my early 30s. The years went by and the gray kept coming in more rapidly, which prompted me to step up my dyeing routine, covering my hair with chemical dyes every 3 weeks. Eventually, not only did gray roots appear after a week, but also my hair started falling at a rapid rate. The harsh chemicals I had been applying for all that time had made my facial skin pale and dull.

The skin around my eyes was dark and dry. I had started taking biotin supplements for more than a year, yet the hair fall did not abate. I started cutting ten inches of my waist length hair to just below my chin. My hair now looked washed-out, dry, frizzy, lackluster and brittle, which was the result of abusing it for years with harsh chemicals.

I was ready for a change. Anjali gave me a shopping list of herbs to buy and instructions on how to apply them to my scalp. After four months of religiously following Anjali's advice and applying her

Ayurvedic remedies, I noticed my hair was falling less and was growing at a faster rate. I also noticed that fresh black hair was coming in with my gray roots. I was actually growing new hair and my hair was getting thicker day by day, week after week.

Ayurveda has changed my life. My hair is at last healthy, shiny, vibrant and long. Even my skin looks better.

This life changing experience has encouraged me to learn more about this ancient art of healing and its power to transform people's lives. I hope that through this book I will be able to transform your life as well. I assure you that not only will your hair stop falling out and start growing back, but you will feel the added side-benefit of a healthier, more vibrant life.

clarifying purposes only and are the owned by the owners themselves, not affiliated with this document.

Chapter 1 - Understanding Hair Loss

Hair loss is a very common condition and can happen to anyone. Being considered to give someone beauty appeal, hair loss can immensely affect not only someone's appearance, but most importantly someone's emotional, psychological and social aspect. Hence, the loss of it could be devastating to a person. It could create a strong negative impact on the overall wellbeing of the person.

There are millions of hair loss sufferers all over the world, comprised of 60% males and 40% females. In a recent study, it was garnered that almost a million hair loss sufferers sought medical treatment to prevent hair loss. There are many treatments that boast of cessation of hair loss and promotion of hair regrowth. However, not all of them are proven to be effective. Ayurveda hair loss remedies have gained worldwide popularity because they are proven safe, all natural and highly successful in treating hair loss and stimulating regrowth.

To better understand why hair loss occurs and how that can be prevented, one should have a thorough understanding of the science of hair and its growth first.

What is hair?

For an average person, the head hair is composed of around one million follicles during the 22nd week in the womb of the mother. This number will be the hair follicles of the individual for the whole lifetime, as hair follicles are not produced anymore after delivery from the womb.

The hair is composed of 2 distinct features:

- Roots – these can be found inside the skin (just under the scalp). Each hair root has a pouch-like structure known as follicle. This pouch has nerve fibers and capillaries.

- Shafts – the strands visible on top of the scalp. It is composed of three layers, with the cuticle at the outermost layer, medulla in the innermost and cortex in between cuticle and medulla.

The hair grows about 6 inches per year. According to statistics, there are about 40-50% women with long hair (up to the shoulder blades). It may not be a surprise that studies revealed that men prefer women with long, straight, flowing hair. Consequently, women feel more feminine and attractive when wearing long hairstyles.

Normally, there is a loss of around 100 strands per 100,000 hair follicles per day. When it is more than this, then it could be alarming. It could lead to gross hair fall resulting to thinning of hair (for women) and development of bald patches (for men). This could be a scary experience for both males and females. Hence, prevention of hair loss and maintenance of healthy hair are the priorities for many.

The causes of abnormal fall and loss of hair can vary from the following factors:

- Heredity
- Underlying medical conditions
- Stress
- Anemia
- Poor diet
- Deficiency in Vitamin B6 and folic acid
- Unclean scalp
- Hormonal imbalance
- Improper or too tight tying of hair

Ayurvedic Beliefs About Hair And its Loss

For Ayurveda, hair is a bi-product of the bone tissue hence it has the same nutrients as the bones. To better understand hair loss as believed by the Ayurvedic principles, one must learn the following terms first.

- <u>Vata</u>. This covers the movements of the mind and body. It is in charge of the blood flow, excretion of body wastes and breathing. It is also responsible for the movement and flow of thoughts across the mind. Since the other two principles are dependent on Vata, it is considered as the leader among the three principles of Ayurveda.
- <u>Pitta</u>. This principle governs the mind's and body's heat, metabolism and transformation. Included in its functions are digestion of food, stimulation of the sensory perceptions and discrimination between right and wrong.
- <u>Kapha</u>. The structure and lubrication of both the mind and body are the responsibilities of Kapha. It controls lubrication of lungs and joints, body weight, and growth. In addition, the formation of the seven tissues namely blood, muscles, fat, bones, reproductive tissues, marrow and nutritive fluids are also under the coverage of the Kapha principle.

The reasons for the hair loss according to Ayurverda are manifold. However the chief reason is excess Pitta Dosha, meaning there is excess heat in the body. The good news is that there are many Ayurveda remedies available to treat and stop hair loss and regrow beautiful, thick hair.

One must take note however that Ayurveda's art of healing is not plain treatment or management of hair loss only. It is a lifestyle. It involves changes in one's activities, diet, thoughts and even feelings. This may sound overwhelming for someone whose purpose is just to stop hair loss but in the long run, one would be able to say that it is all worth it.

Your goal may be just to prevent further hair thinning or to have your beautiful, thick hair back but following the Ayurveda remedies would do more than that for you. It also affects your mind, will and emotions positively. You will come out of this therapy physically, emotionally, psychologically and even spiritually healthy. You will come out a changed person.

Are you ready to say goodbye to hair thinning, baldness, and hair loss and say hello to shiny, healthy, strong hair through the

Ayurveda hair loss remedies? Do you want to be healthier, fitter, lighter, and more energetic? Do you want peace and serenity of your mind and heart, too? Then read on. This book will bring your hair back plus so much more!

Chapter 2 - Ayurvedic Dietary Program To Combat Hair Loss

The primary reason for hair loss could be traced to excess Pitta Dosha in the body. Hence the solution is to avoid having that excess. This is easily remedied by having a dietary regimen that would eliminate or lessen consumption of those foods that encourage increase or production of excess heat in the body.

Healthy locks would just be one benefit of this diet and for hair loss victims, this benefit is more than enough. There is more to it than this though. In the course of following the dietary suggestions, one would end up leaner, stronger and healthier also. Many followers of the diet have opted to continue with the regimen even when the hair problem is solved already. That is indeed a wise decision. As mentioned, this should become a lifestyle and not just a temporary treatment.

One thing you would notice is that the Ayurveda diet is easy to do. The dishes are easy to prepare, affordable and available in local grocery stores. They taste great, too. One can also start an indoor container gardening of some of the ingredients. These herbs and plants are low maintenance plus truly beneficial to one's overall health.

Foods to take

Here are the recommended foods to consume with the Ayurveda Diet. These foods are rich in Vitamins C and B complex, important fatty acids, zinc and sulfur, which are known to make the roots of the hair really strong.

- High protein foods such as:
    - Soya bean
    - Milk
    - Cheese
    - Butter

- Buttermilk
- Ghee
- Seeds
- Grains
- Nuts
- Yogurt
- Seasonal vegetables and fruits (especially those that contain high fiber)
  - Sprouts made from Chana dal or Moong

Part of the regimen is drinking 10 and more glasses of water every day. Doing this cleanses the body from accumulated toxins and wastes.

Foods to avoid

These foods can aggravate Pitta and cause increase heat to the body.

- Spicy foods
- Fried or greasy foods
- Sour foods
- Meats
- White flour (pastries, bread, pasta, etc.)
- White sugar
- Junk foods (chips, candies, processed foods etc.)
- Foods with artificial colors and preservatives
- Excess intake of the following (you may consume these but in moderation)
  - Tea
  - Coffee
  - Pickles
  - Alcohol

On top of these, try to do the following recommended recipes and dishes to aid hair regrowth and stop hair loss.

- Drink 1/3 cup of aloe vera juice once a day or make a concoction of 1 tablespoon aloe vera gel and a pinch of cumin to be taken three times a day for 3 months. This has been effective in controlling and combatting hair fall. Watch out for diarrhea, as this is the side effect of aloe vera when taken in excess. Follow the recommended dosage only.

- Drinking fresh juices made from alfalfa, carrots, lettuce and spinach will aid hair regrowth.
- Add a spoonful of sesame seeds (white) every day to your breakfast. Sesame seeds are a great source of calcium and magnesium. These are the nutrients vital to bone health (remember for Ayurveda, hair needs the same nutrients as bones).
- Known to reduce hair fall and thinning to a large extent is the consumption of yogurt on a daily basis. Plus, yogurt contains good bacteria beneficial to the digestive system.
- Have large servings of high fiber fruits and vegetables to prevent constipation. When there is good bowel movement, the health of the hair also improves.

The Ayurvedic diet guarantees stronger and healthier hair and prevention and control of hair fall. Try it today.

Chapter 3 - Ayurvedic Hair Loss Cure

Ayurvedic remedies for hair loss make great use of different herbs. These herbs are available in local grocery stores or you can order them online, such as Amazon.com. Planting them in pots or containers is recommended so that you will have a steady supply of these herbs at any time.

Below are several effective herbal treatments you can use to prevent hair loss and to regrow new hair.

1. *Use of Bhringaraj (King of Herbs)*

To enhance hair growth and arrest premature graying of hair, make a paste out of fresh Bhringaraj (also known as false daisy or Eclipta alba) leaves. Apply on the scalp and leave it there for 15 to 30 minutes. Rinse with water. In case fresh leaves are not available, use a pack of dried Bhringaraj, which can be ordered on Amazon.com. Simply steep these dried leaves in warm water (around 5-6 tablespoons), apply on the scalp and wash off after the designated time. If you perform this routine on a regular basis you will notice plenty of new hair growth within just a few months.

2. *Use of lemon juice and Indian gooseberry*

Simply cut the Indian gooseberry (also known as Amla or Amlaki) into smaller pieces and remove the seeds. Crush the pieces until they become a paste. Strain the paste so that the juice can be extracted. Use a sieve (wire or plastic mesh) to do this. Add 3 tablespoons of lemon juice to the extracted juice of Indian gooseberry. Mix very well. Apply the mixture to the scalp and leave on for 30 minutes. After the recommended time, wash the hair with water.

Another variation is the use of dried or powdered Indian gooseberry, available on Amazon.com. Mix it with warm water and apply on the scalp. Rinse off after 15 minutes.

3. *Hair loss natural home remedy using lemon peel, soap nut, curry leaves, green gram and fenugreek seeds*

Gather the following ingredients and place in one container:

- 1 lemon peel
- 3 tablespoons of soap nut powder
- 15-20 pieces of curry leaves
- 2 tablespoons of green gram
- 2 tablespoons of fenugreek seeds

Grind the ingredients. Place the mixture into a clean, glass bottle. Use this mixture as your shampoo. Rinse well with water.

4. *Use of Margosa leaves*

Crush a handful of margosa leaves and add to a pot filled with 4 cups of water. Bring to a boil. Allow the liquid to cool and filter out the leaves. Use this liquid when rinsing your hair.

5. *Use of Aromatic Jatamansi*

This herb root goes by the names of Indian Spikenard and Muskroot. It aids in stimulating hair growth by removing blood impurities. It is also known for causing the skin to glow radiantly. It is available in capsule forms. You can either take the capsule orally (not more than 6 mgs per day) or apply it directly on the scalp.

6. *Use of Methi (Miracle Herb)*

Another great remedy for hair growth is Methi, or better known as Fenugreek. Choose the dry roasted methi and grind it. Add in warm water and make a paste out of it. Apply on scalp and hair. Leave it on for 20 minutes then wash off with water.

7. *Other Herbs*

Trichup herbal hair powder or THHP is a mixture of the following herbs: bhringaraj, brahmi, Indian gooseberry, aloe vera, henna, neem, and jatamansi. THHP is used for treating split ends and dandruff and preventing hair fall. Another herb is Teak wood seed extracts. This herb promotes hair growth.

Some Thoughts on the Use of Herbs

Today's shampoos, conditioners and other hair products are found to be harsh both on the scalp and hair strands. The above mentioned herbal remedies use all natural ingredients and herbs that are not only safe and healthy to your scalp and hair but also friendly to the environment.

Chapter 4 - Ayurvedic Oils and Massage

Massaging the head is the act of applying pressure on the scalp using the fingers and hands. Ayurvedic massage makes use of techniques involving kneading and rubbing, which promotes increased blood flow to the scalp. With adequate tissue perfusion, nutrients and oxygen are delivered to the hair follicles, making them strong and healthy, thus preventing hair loss.

Adding oil during the head massage has proven to be beneficial. The oil nourishes the hair and scalp. It promotes hair growth by reducing the conditions that cause hair fall such as dry scalp, dandruff, brittle hair and split ends.

Here are the recommended oils to use during head massage according to the Ayurveda system of healing.

- *Bhringaraj*

The King of herbs can also be combined with coconut or sesame oil to be used as oil during a scalp massage or as hair dressing during regular days. This mixture is rich in protein, a vital ingredient in making the hair strong and healthy. As a welcome side effect, Bhringaraj can also restore the original color of the hair.

- *Brahmi*

Also known as Gotu Kola, Water hyssop and Indian Pennywort, Brahmi is a herb that can be mixed with a base oil like sesame oil to prevent premature hair loss. It also helps to thicken the hair and add volume to it. Another benefit is its calming effects on the mind and nervous system.

- *Almond Oil*

For hair that is frizzy, thin, dry and prone to have split ends, Almond oil is recommended. Whether in its pure form or as carrier of other Ayurvedic oils, it will add luster, strength and shine to the hair as well as control loss of hair. Why? Almond oil is very rich in Vitamin E, Calcium and Magnesium.

- *Coconut Oil*

Coconut oil is effective for fine hair. This type of hair is susceptible to thinning and premature graying. According to studies made, coconut oil can delay the hair-shedding process. Coconut Oil is also used as carrier oil to amalaki and other ayurvedic oils.

- *Sesame Oil*

Loaded with manganese, copper, calcium, Vitamin B1, this oil is used for frizzy, dry hair. In addition, it has antifungal, antibacterial and antioxidant properties. Sesame oil head and hair massage is highly recommended for those who regularly swim in pools as it can protect the hair from chlorine.

- *Neem Seed Oil*

Also called Azadica Indica, Neem seed oil is packed with essential fatty acids and Vitamin E. It possesses antiviral, antibacterial and antifungal properties. This oil is combined with olive oil.

- *Amalaki Oil (Indian Gooseberry)*

Also called Amla, this oil is effective for thick and oily hair. It is rich in Vitamin C, polyphenols, tannins, and flavonoids. It rejuvenates the hair and prevents premature graying.

- *Final Words on Ayurvedic Oils*

Other medicated Ayurvedic oils for hair growth are Mahabhringraj oil and Arnica oil. Regular massaging of head and hair can stimulate increased blood flow leading to healthier hair roots. Within 6 months, thicker and lustrous hair will be noticeable. Continue to massage with medicated Ayurvedic oils even after six months for maintenance of hair health.

Chapter 5 - Ayurveda Lifestyle: A Cure For Hair Loss

The Ayurvedic lifestyle, or Dinacharya, came from the combined words "Din" meaning day and "acharya" meaning to follow. It literally means to follow in a day or a better translation is routine or daily regimen. The Ayurveda principle believes that in order for a person to achieve optimal health, healthy living/lifestyle must be a part of one's daily schedule.

This also applies to having healthy hair. Your diet should become a healthy routine of eating plenty of fresh food, such as vegetables, fruit and legumes and drinking plenty of fresh water. The above recommended massages with medicated oils should be performed regularly. Hair hygienic practices using herbal ingredients should become a daily routine. Ayurveda is not a one-time treatment. It is a lifestyle ensuring health and vitality.

Aside from the abovementioned lifestyle modifications, here are other things I recommend that you observe to guarantee not only prevention of hair loss but also a total sense of wellbeing.

1. Cessation of smoking. Hundreds of studies have linked cigarette smoking (specifically its nicotine content) to various medical disorders. Smoking can damage the hair because it causes constriction of vessels, making it more difficult for the blood to flow. This decreases the supplies of nutrients and oxygen to the hair follicles.
2. Stress management. Stress affects the overall wellbeing of the person. Physically, aside from hair loss, one can experience palpitation, shortness of breath, dry mouth and skin, disruption of the digestive system, headache, and other symptoms. Stress can also cause mental fatigue, emotional instability, anxiety, sleep disturbance, poor appetite, and poor decision making skills. It affects one's social life too. A

stressed person tends to withdraw himself from others. In addition, that would also affect his performance either in school or work. Therefore, it is vital that a person knows how to manage stress. There are many relaxation techniques that one can practice. Below I have listed recommended Ayurvedic stress management techniques that will not only prevent hair loss and ensure hair regrowth, but also maintain the overall health of the individual.

    a. Yoga. This is divided into three types, according to the three Ayurvedic principles, which are vata, pitta and kapha (discussed in Chapter 1)

        i. For Vata, the recommended yoga would include meditative practice, Tadasana or mountain pose, Paschimittanasana (seated forward bend), Vrkasana (tree pose) and halasana (plow pose).

        ii. For Pitta, mild, restorative yoga that includes Baddha konasana (bound Angle Pose), Paschimittanasana (seated forward bend), and Janu Sirasana (a head-to-knee- pose).

        iii. For Kapha, the recommended yoga is heat producing with vigorous movement. Included in this are backbends, sun salutations, chest-opening poses such as Ustrasana or Camel pose and Dhanurasana or Bow pose.

    b. Aromatherapy and healing herbs.

        i. For Vata – cardamom, cinnamon and ginger

        ii. For Pitta – Rose, jasmine and lavender

        iii. For Kapha – Frankincense and Rosemary

    c. Deep breathing exercise

3. Have adequate rest and sleep. The body needs to rejuvenate and recharge itself. It can do this when the person rests and sleeps. The hair greatly benefits from this healthy lifestyle as the cells of the hair follicles are repaired or reproduced during resting and sleeping periods.

4. Limiting alcoholic beverages. Alcohol has been linked to numerous medical ailments. A social drink of 1-2 glasses a

week is tolerable. However, daily consumption can be hazardous to your hair and of course, your overall health.

5. Daily bowel movement. The accumulation of wastes and toxins in the body greatly contributes to hair loss. Therefore, expulsion of these wastes will result in radiant hair. A person should have at least one bowel movement a day. It should be soft and well-formed, easy to pass and not foul smelling. If you are constipated, harmful toxins build up inside of your body. To fight constipation, increase your fiber and water intake and physical activity. I highly recommend a juicing routine (see book recommendation in Appendix). Having diarrhea may seem better than constipation but it is actually just as harmful. Diarrhea can lead to poor absorption of essential nutrients. Having a regular, healthy bowel movement is the ideal scenario for a healthy life. A healthy gut is a healthy person. It was Hippocrates over 2000 years ago who believed that all diseases start in the gut.

6. Avoiding too much direct sun exposure and other heat-causing agents. Pitta dosha or excess heat in the body can cause hair loss, according to Ayurveda belief. Therefore, one must avoid foods that can cause elevation of heat of the body. Maintain a cool body by staying indoors or avoiding the harsh direct sunlight. During summer, wear clothes made of light material and color. In addition, increase the fluid intake to refresh the body and replenish fluid losses. Avoid saunas and other warm places.

Having a healthy lifestyle is a major factor in having beautiful, full head of hair. Listen to your body, mind and heart. As you follow the Ayurvedic lifestyle, you will not only look more attractive (because of your shiny and lustrous hair) but also be more radiant, healthy and happy, which is the most important aspect in someone's life.

Chapter 6 - Inner Peace Equals Healthy Hair

A lot of people may wonder what the connection between inner tranquility and healthy hair is. Ayurveda is all about balance between the body, soul and spirit. When the innermost being of the person is calm and at peace, the mind and body relaxes and experiences calmness, too. When there is inner peace, there is a healthy spirit and in return a healthy mind and body.

Achieving inner peace is vital in order to have healthy hair. However, aside from preventing hair loss and growing thick, healthy hair, inner peace will give you contentment, joy, happiness and a sense of fulfillment like no other.

How does one achieve inner peace? Here are secrets to having inner peace.

1. **Meditation**. Having a quiet time for reflection and pondering can help calm your mind and spirit. We are living in a very busy and stressed culture. Everybody is constantly rushing. There are deadlines, traffic, numerous activities, and responsibilities. Enjoying a few minutes just thinking of positive and wonderful things can boost tranquility and serenity in your life. Allot time for this every day in your schedule.
2. **Practicing Yoga**. The word yoga actually means to unite the body, mind and spirit. Hence, it comes as a no surprise that Yoga benefits the body, mind and spirit. Enroll in a class or do yoga exercises at home.
3. **Doing spiritual activities** like praying, reading spiritual books, singing, and attending retreats or conventions. I recommended a healthy diet in order to strengthen your physical body. Now I am recommending a diet for your spirit, which is equally important. You have to nourish your mind, body and spirit in order to be a healthy, well-balanced individual with inner peace.

4. **Forgiveness**. Carrying with you the heavy burdens of not being able to forgive the wrongs of others will just backfire on you. Let go of the past and move forward.
5. **Doing special things to others**. When your focus is lifted from yourself and you begin to care and be of service to others, you are actually doing yourself a favor. There is joy in being able to assist others, especially those who have no way of returning the favor to you. Volunteer for charity works. Give to the poor and needy. Look around and try to be of help to others around you, whether they are friends or strangers.
6. **Being grateful**. Taking the time to appreciate what you have will give you the peace that you are longing for. Look at your family and be thankful that you have a family. Look at your surroundings. There are many things to be grateful about if you just took time to look for them. Learn to count your blessings rather than your failures.
7. **Breath properly**. Proper breathing is one key to a clear and peaceful mind. At least 2-3 times a day, take note of your respiration. Take deep breaths slowly through the mouth. Hold the breath for 5 seconds. Release or exhale through the nose and mouth and then repeat the process again. This simple activity is very helpful in calming the nerves and relaxing the whole body.
8. **Smile**. This simple gesture will not only delight the recipients but also improve your overall well-being. Smiling improves the circulation and releases certain hormones and enzymes in the body, giving you extra energy.

Health is holistic. It is not just about the physical aspect. It is all encompassing. Ayurveda is highly successful in treating hair loss because its remedies are focused on the totality of the individual and not only on one single aspect.

Hair is one of the best gauges to determine how healthy a person really is. Today, enjoy shiny, strong and healthy hair with Ayurvedic remedies for hair loss. Make it a lifestyle and you will find yourself enjoying a healthy body, mind and spirit.

Conclusion

Thank you again for purchasing this book.

I am certain that, if you apply the Ayurvedic remedies described in this book, you will experience a total body and life transformation. Stopping your hair loss and growing back healthy, shiny hair will be a wonderful added benefit to your complete health of mind, body and spirit.

The cure is in your hands. Now it is up to you to take action and implement life changes that only you can control. Most importantly, stay determined and focus on the new Ayurvedic routines, diet and lifestyle until these new routines become your everyday habits.

Lastly, if you enjoyed reading this book, I would greatly appreciate your kind book reviews on Amazon.com. I am especially looking forward to reading your success stories of how Ayurveda helped stop your hair loss and transformed your life into radiant health and beauty.

Appendix

Preview of 'GMO Free Diet: The Ultimate Guide on Avoiding GMO Foods and keeping Your Family Healthy with a GMO Free Diet'

Chapter 1- GMOs: The Big No-No!

Genetically Modified Organisms (or GMOs) have swept the world of consumption and biotechnology industry in a very controversial manner. The term itself has prompted several countries to ban their production. Many skeptical consumers have likewise challenged state laws in making GMO labeling mandatory in all food products sold on the market.

BUT the question is – what really are these so-called GMOs?

To quote World Health Organization's definition: "GMOs are organisms in which the genetic material (DNA) has been altered in a way that does not occur naturally".

As the name suggests, GMOs are 'genetically engineered' foods or crops. The genetic makeup of these foods is modified or manipulated artificially through validated genetic engineering process. The process has created a range of produce, which are engineered so as to control characteristics such as disease resistance, pesticide resistance, herbicide resistance, nutritional content, and even ripening. Thus, this is a new science that evidently produces 'unstable' bacteria and viruses that could never be produced through natural methods. To put simply, GMOs are 'manipulated' to confer certain traits that are not natural for the organism.

Commercial GMOs have anchored their way on the global market through enticing promises which include:

- Increased yield

- Climate-change ready crops

- Reduced need for the use of pesticides and/or herbicides

- Improved nutrition content of the crops compared to naturally grown produce

- Reduced risks of food shortage

On the other hand, with the growing popularity of GMOs come a range of issues connected to environmental damages and health problems, as well as the violation of farmers' rights and consumer's rights.

So how did GMOs break into the global market?

The transfer of DNA from one organism to another was found possible and viable back in 1946. However, the real application took place roughly four decades after this discovery. The first ever recorded genetically modified/engineered plant came about in 1983, when a tobacco plant was made anti-biotic resistant.

In 1994, The Food and Drug Administration in the US approved the sale of 'Flavr Savr' tomato, the first food-related genetically modified organism. The company, Calgene in California, started to produce this tomato variant using genetically engineered seeds that have been injected with ACC synthase. Such gene allows ripening to take place after the tomatoes have been picked manually. This particular product has also become a catalyst for the production of more GMOs- particularly the BT corn, BT potato, and canola. Glyphosate (herbicide) –resistant squash followed suit. In 2010, another GMO breakthrough was recorded when scientists were able to augment the Vitamin A content of rice. This rice variant has been on the commercial market ever since.

To read more and purchase this book go to http://amzn.to/1DEKJVz

Other Book Recommendations:

Juicing for Health: The Essential Guide To Healing Common Diseases with Proven Juicing Recipes and Staying Healthy For Life by Donna Cavanaugh

The Auto Immune Solution: Learn how to Prevent and Overcome Inflammatory Diseases and Live a Pain-Free Life by Anthony Weil

Clean Gut: The Breakthrough Plan for Eliminating the Root Cause of Disease and Revolutionizing Your Health by Alejandro Junger

Cannabis Oil Cures: How to cure cancer for life, improve health immediately, lose weight within 30 days and look younger with Cannabis Oil by Michael Skinner

"Edible Wild Plants for Beginners: The Essential Edible Plants and Recipes to Get Started" by Athea Press

On My Own Two Feet: From Losing My Legs to Learning the Dance of Life by Amy Purdy

Living and Dealing with Crazy People: The Ultimate Guide On How To Make Your Life Crazy-Proof by Michael Skinner

Become the next American Ninja Warrior: The Ultimate Guide on How to Prepare and Win the next American Ninja Warrior Obstacle Race by Brian Davidson

Other Book Recommendations:

...

www.ingramcontent.com/pod-product-compliance
Lightning Source LLC
Chambersburg PA
CBHW070942290526
45795CB00003B/1122